Ketogenic Diet

14 Day step by step beginners guide to a high fat, low carbohydrates diet to lose weight and feel amazing.

Table of Contents

Introduction

It could be that you are planning to go on a Keto Diet! But before taking that step, you should first try to educate yourself as to what it is all about. It is only a thorough research, proper understanding and well-informed decision that can help you to get the desired results. At the same time, you will be able to avoid the issues and side effects (if any involved).

What is ketogenic diet?

The keto diet is considered to be low carb diet. Here, the body is required to produce within the liver, "ketones" for using it as energy. There are several names attributed to it like LCHF (low - carb high fat), low carb diet, ketogenic diet, etc.

If you consume food that is high in carbs, then your body will start to produce insulin and glucose.

- For processing glucose within your bloodstream, insulin is produced. It is achieved by absorbing it across the body.
- The easiest molecule is Glucose for the body to convert, to be used as energy. This way, it can be selected over the other types of energy source.

As glucose is used as primary energy, there is no need for fats and hence get stored. On the normal, typically, the higher carbohydrate diet, where glucose is used by the body as the main energy form. It is by reducing carbohydrate intake that the body gets induced into a particular state called ketosis.

Ketosis is regarded to be a natural process which is initiated by the body. It is done to help people to survive if intake of food is found to be low. It is during this state that ketones are produced, achieved through the breakdown of fats within the liver.

There is a need to maintain keto diet and its objective is to compel the body to be in this metabolic state. This is not done through calorie starvation, but via carbohydrate starvation.

Whatever is being put inside the body, it is able to adapt to it incredibly. When it is overloaded with fats and have the carbohydrates taken away, then it is likely to burn up the ketones as a primary source of energy. The optimal levels of ketone are likely to offer weight loss, health, mental and physical performance benefits.

More about Keto Diet

In a nutshell, the ketogenic diet can be termed to be adequate protein, high fat, low carbohydrate diet. It is used in medicine for treating primarily refractory epilepsy noticed among small children and is difficult to control. The body burns up fats instead of carbohydrates when this diet is practiced. Generally, glucose is transported throughout the body and is considered to be crucial for fueling better brain function. With little carbohydrate being present within the diet, fat is converted by the liver into ketone bodies and fatty acids. Ketone bodies then pass into the brain, to replace the glucose as the primary energy source. Epileptic seizures decline in frequency with the ketone bodies being found in elevated level within the blood.

The therapeutic diet that is originally provided for pediatric epilepsy offers sufficient protein for repair and growth of the body. Also, calories in necessary amount are provided for maintaining correct weight related to height and age. Such classic ketogenic diet is known to contain fat weight to combined carbohydrate and protein by a ratio of 4:1. It is achieved by having high carbohydrate foods excluded like starchy fruits, bread, vegetables, sugar, grains, and pasta. At the same time, it demands increasing consumption of foods that are rich in fats like butter, cream, and nuts. The majority of the dietary fat is created from molecules known as LCTs (long chain triglycerides). But MCTs (medium chain triglycerides) created from fatty acids along with short carbon chains when compared to LCTs are considered to be more ketogenic. MCT ketogenic diet, a classic diet variant is said to use a coconut oil type that has plenty of MCTs in it. This offers about half the calories. Since this diet variant requires less overall fat, a good proportion of protein and carbohydrate is likely to be consumed, thereby allowing greater food choice and variety.

Increasing popularity

It is for treating pediatric epilepsy that therapeutic ketogenic diet had been developed during the 1920s. It was used widely even in the next decade. However, with the effective anticonvulsant drug being introduced, its popularity started to wane. During the mid-1990s, Jim Abrahams, the popular Hollywood producer, whose son was suffering from severe epilepsy, got cured completely of this diet. For promoting this miracle diet, he had started the Charlie Foundation. The publicity that was launched for the promotion of this diet included an appearance on Dateline program of NBC as well as a movie made for the television starring Meryl Streep named "First Do No Harm" released in 1997.

A multi-centre research study was sponsored by the foundation. It was in 1996 that its results had been announced, which marked the start of the renewed scientific interest shown in this particular diet.

People with epilepsy, which comprised about half of the children as well as young people had at first tried out some kind of this diet. They found that the seizure numbers dropped considerably by about half. The effect was noticed to persist even though the diet was discontinued. Constipation was noticed to be the common adverse effect that is said to have affected around 30% of the patients. It is because of fluid restriction that once was a specific feature of the keto diet. It has led to enhanced risk of developing kidney stones. Thus, it is no longer stated to be beneficial. Some evidence is found that adults suffering from epilepsy might benefit from consuming this diet. Again, following a less stringent regimen like the modified Atkins diet is also found to be effective. Clinical studies and trials in the animal models, which include C. Elegans, have suggested that disease modifying and neuroprotective benefits for several adult neurodegenerative disorders. The limited clinical trial had been conducted and data found in these areas as well as external of pediatric epilepsy. Thus, using the ketogenic diet is said to remain at the research stage.

Its history

This diet is actually a mainstream therapy which does not make use of pharmaceutical drugs. It has been developed for the purpose of reproducing the success as well as removal of existing limitations of non-mainstream usage of fasting for treating epilepsy. Even though it became popular during the 1920s & 30s, this was abandoned largely favoring new anticonvulsant drugs. With proper and timely medication, it became possible for individuals with epilepsy to control successfully their seizures. But 20% to 30% of the people tend to fail in achieving control despite different drugs are being tried out. For this particular group, especially for children, the diet has found a particular role within epilepsy management.

Chapter 1
Why should you opt for a ketogenic diet?

By opting for keto diet, it is possible to derive several benefits. Some of the benefits enjoyed are increased levels of energy, to weight loss to therapeutic medical applications. It is possible for anyone to benefit immensely from consuming high fat, low carb diet.

- Weight loss: Such type of diet is likely to make use of the body fat as a source of energy. There are obvious benefits of weight loss, something that cannot be simply denied. Your insulin levels (the hormone which stores fat) on keto tends to drop immensely, thereby turning the body into a fat burning machine. Ketogenic diet scientifically is seen to display much better results when compared to high carb and low-fat diets even during the longer term period. Any person planning to incorporate MCT oil within his diet (to increase production of ketone and witness fat loss) should drink in the morning ketoprofen coffee.

- Helps control level of blood sugar: Blood sugar levels lowers down naturally through keto diet because of the food type consumed. According to studies, the ketogenic diet has been found to be a much effective way towards managing as well as preventing diabetes when compared to those low-calorie diets. In case, you are suffering from Type 2 diabetes or are pre-diabetic, then it is necessary on your part to take into consideration a ketogenic diet. People in huge numbers have been noticed to have experienced the success in controlling their blood sugar level by availing keto diet.

- Normalized hunger and increased energy: You are likely to get more energized throughout the day by providing your body with a much more reliable and better source of energy. Fats are undoubtedly quite an effective molecule that can burn well as fuel. Besides this, fat is noticed to be much more satisfying naturally and keep us in a much more "full" (satiated) state for a longer time period.
- Mental focus: Ketogenic diet is used by many people especially to enjoy increased mental performance. For the brain, ketones do make a fabulous fuel source. Upon lowering down intake of carb, the big spikes noticed in blood sugar can be prevented. Combined together, it may result in enhanced concentration and focus. According to studies, increased consumption of fatty acids is likely to have a positive impact on the brain's functions.
- Blood pressure and cholesterol: Cholesterol levels and triglyceride levels are seen to be improved with a keto diet. They are associated mostly with arterial buildup. The dramatic increase is found in HDL along with the reduction of LDL particle concentration when compared to low-fat diets in high fat, low carb diets. Better improvement has been found in blood pressure when compared to the other diets according to studies conducted on low-carb diets. Excess weight does create issues related to blood pressure. It is actually a bonus as keto leads towards loss of weight.

- Epilepsy: It is right from the early 1900s that ketogenic diet is found to help treat successfully epilepsy. Still, it is regarded to be among the most widely utilized therapies especially among children today experiencing uncontrolled epilepsy. A major benefit derived from this type of diet is that fewer medications are allowed to be used. Still, it offers you with excellent control. Studies conducted during the last few years have shown that adults who were treated with keto had displayed significant results.

- Insulin resistance: Resistance to insulin is likely to lead towards the development of type 2 diabetes, especially when it is left unmanaged. Research performed in this area has shown clearly that low carb diet can assist people to reduce their levels of insulin to healthy ranges. Even if the person is athletic, he/she can still benefit from availing insulin optimization upon keto, which is achieved through consumptions of foods that are high in Omega Three fatty acids.

- Acne: Upon switching to ketogenic diet, you are likely to experience skin improvements which are termed to be a common factor. Studies have confirmed there has been a drastic reduction in skin inflammation and lesions when low carb diet is being followed. Other studies conducted show probable connection n between increased acne and high carb consumption. It is here that keto can prove to be of great help. For acne, it can prove to be beneficial for reducing intake of dairy products and to follow stringent skin cleaning regimen.

- Treatment of diseases: Even though it is primarily used for treating epilepsy, reduction in carbohydrate intake can boost drastically level of metabolism in your body. This not only leads towards loss of weight but also in elimination or amelioration of diseases. Such diets have been helpful for treating cardiovascular diseases. This is achieved by lowering down cholesterol levels, pumping blood lipid panels. This diet also is noticed to be helpful to treat type two diabetes. This is done by reducing resistance to insulin and glucose outputs.

- Low carb brain fuel: A major aspect with regards to ketogenic diet is regarded to be the kind of benefit that it offers to the human brain. It is by increasing ketone circulation in the body, stronger and better fuel gets pumped within the brain. This, in turn, leads to increased energy and focus. At the same time, it also helps to prevent and treat multiple neurological disorders.

- Eliminate glucose that forces burning of fat in the body: Ketogenic diet's objective is to compel the body to enter Ketosis. It effectively means that rather than relying upon glucose, which is developed with the breakdown of carbohydrates for providing the body with sufficient fuel to energize ourselves, the body is regarded to search for ways to use stored fat for energizing the body and the mind. As the essential carbohydrate amount required for converting into energy gets restricted, those materials are found by the body from other sources present. With a whole new metabolism method being created, it tends to serve as a jump start to prevent weight. But, people who are advised to go on a ketogenic diet are required to work out regularly for the desired effects to set in. This is proven to be much more beneficial when compared to performing only the exercise.

- Effects of ketogenic diets upon cellular energy: Ketogenic diet also has found to be successful to create a positive impact upon the body cells. It is already understood that increased ketone circulation can prove the brain with more energy. It effectively means that ketones are likely to increase in brain cell numbers themselves. Besides this, such new and improvised brain cells are said to contain mitochondria, stated to be the cells' powerhouse. They are packed with very high energy levels along with an increase in productivity, due to the presence of ketones. It leads towards increased energy levels as well as feelings of alertness. It is stated to be responsible towards an increase in the production of metabolism and burning stored fat. It is due to these factors that ketogenic diet is noticed to helping in improvising the overall brain function and assist with memory loss.
- Can help safeguard against Cancer: There is no 100% guarantee that by adopting this type of diet will remove all possibilities of cancer. It has been shown by researchers that increased functioning of the brain combined with medication is effective to reduce the cancerous brain tumors. Again ketogenic diet, when used along with radiation therapy, can help to eliminate completely brain tumor cells. The diet's success related to helping patients with cancers and tumors is because of the diet's limitation with respect to growth factor stimulation. This does mean that the growth of the tumor can be limited or stopped all of a sudden. At the same time, it also may assist to prevent inflammation that surrounds the tumor region that again might lead towards a reduction in tumor size and the intense pain that comes with it. It is definitely crucial to

13

stress that on its own, this type of diet will not be able to safeguard against cancer or cure completely the tumors that exist within the body. But, it has been found to be useful when used along with other types of treatments, to reduce pain, speed up the recovery process, to diminish cancerous size as well as that of malign tumors.

- Antioxidants and its power: As ketogenic diet is said to be very high in antioxidants, it has been proved by studies that it helps to avoid oxidative damage that might occur at the time of hypoglycemia. This diet also helps to avoid destruction of the weaker cells besides creating much stronger, newer ones for fighting back disease and infections. The increase of antioxidants within the body is likely to counterbalance the free radical amount present within the body. If the latter is found to be out of balance, then it is likely to lead towards reduced immune system and decreased energy levels. As free radicals are eliminated from the bloodstream, it is not just the immune system getting boosted up, but also there is noticed improving the memory function, strengthening of the eye muscles, and amelioration of the memory and mood issues.

So, it can be safely stated that although ketogenic diet is being practiced for over hundreds of years now, for treating diseases, the success of this diet is what has led to its increasing popularity and demand across the globe. Adopting ketogenic diet and combining it with regular exercise is sure to lead towards the long-term, dramatic success. It is actually by improving the brain function, finding newer ways for creating energy, forcing burning up of fat by the body, reducing carbohydrate consumption and increasing fat intake in the body that this type of diet comes with a multitude of benefits. At the same time, it is completely safe for any person to follow this diet without any kind of side effect or medical issue.

Chapter 2
The 14-day plan

There are many of you whose New Year Resolution probably may have been about losing weight and to become slim and trim as fast as possible but without the side effects. If this is what you have in mind, then this diet plan is sure to bring plenty of inspiration and motivate you to feel great throughout the year and to consume healthily.

Doing some research will help you to come across a complete list of the available free diet plans that you can follow depending on your specific needs, requirements, moods and taste. There are readily available several diet plans that can be followed by anyone like paleo/keto, primal/keto, vegetarian/keto diet plans, along with meal plan to reduce fat quickly! However, all diet plans do include easy to prepare recipes and shopping list. This way, you can ensure not having to waste your precious time in the kitchen and can get your diet plan ready within minutes.

But, before getting into the new diet plan, there are few frequently asked questions that you need to know about keto diet. This way, you can be better prepared to implement them without any hassle or worry.

Tips to get started

- In case, you are the cook, then have the remaining servings refrigerated or frozen or probably get the recipes halved if required.
- You can have breakfast swapped for lunch, lunch for dinner and the like on the same day. At the same

time, you can also have whole days swapped, if you feel like.

- The keto buns are to be made much in advance (full 10 recipes can be prepared). Freeze for keeping fresh as well as defrost the night before at room temperature or in the oven before serving.
- No snacks are to be had in between the meals. In case, you do, then ensure that some keto friendly snacks are consumed.

Given below is some list of snacks that you can try out. Also, is provided a complete list of keto diet food.

- Quite low carb diets (that are below 3 gms of net carbs). These are often devoid in magnesium. Magnesium supplements are recommended or snacks that are high in magnesium are to be included like nuts. If you experience any 'keto flu' symptoms, then ensure consuming additional sodium (like pink Himalayan salt).
- The diet plan probably might not suit every person. In such a case, minor adjustments have to be made. If less protein is desired, then the portions of eggs and meat are to be reduced. Simply leave alone your worries with regards to the small protein excess present, as it would not eliminate you out of ketosis. As a matter of fact, protein is likely to keep your hunger at bay. In case, more or less fat is desired, then you can focus on including fatty foods and oils while making the adjustments. The ideal macros can be found by using Keto Diet buddy!
- Few recipes are found to be much higher in total fiber and carbs. In case, you are of the opinion that your weight loss will be impaired by fiber, then you need to check out what counts really, Net Carbs or

Total Carbs. According to studies, fiber is good for losing weight.

- Avoid eating anything, if you feel full and not hungry. It also will mean skipping a meal.

Chapter 3
How to execute it?

Ketogenic diets and more specifically the Cyclic Ketogenic Diets have been termed to be more effective diets to achieve ultra low, rapid body fat levels combined with optimum muscle retention. There are, however, some circumstantial exceptions. If they are performed right, which are considered to be quite rare, the loss of fat that is achievable with this diet can be stated to be quite staggering! At the same time, you are also likely to enjoy and experience incredible high energy along with overall well being.

Perception

However, it has been noticed that despite such assurances, there are several body builders who have had experienced negative effects instead of positive ones. Some of the main criticisms have been given below:

- Unbearable hunger
- Chronic lethargy
- Severe muscle loss
- Huge decrease noticed in gym performance

The above criticisms are noticed to be the result of a failure for not heeding the above caveat that ketogenic diets are to be performed correctly! There is a genuine need to realize the fact that they are rather a completely unique metabolic modality which tends not to adhere to any of the previously accepted dieting 'rules'. Also, there is no point in going half way. The truth is having carbs about 50 grams in a day along with high protein intake *cannot* be termed as ketogenic.

Therefore, the question is how to get the ketogenic diet performed correctly? Check out below how they work.

Ketosis and its overview

Ketones or glucose can be used as fuel by our brain, muscles, organs and the entire body. This fuel supply is regulated primarily by the pancreas and the liver. They tend to show a very strong bias for sticking with glucose. The latter is considered to be the 'preferred' fuel. This is due to the fact that it is found in plenty from this diet and is available readily from muscle stores and the liver. the liver is required to synthesize deliberately the ketones. However, glucose can be synthesized easily by the liver through a process called 'gluconeogenesis', which makes use of amino acids (protein). It can also use any other metabolic intermediaries.

From this diet, acetoacetate (ketones), acetone or hydroxybutyrate is not derived. They are synthesized by the liver only under duress. It is rather performed as the last measure during conditions of severe deprivation of glucose such as starvation. In order to convince the liver that ketones are crucial for the body, there are several conditions which are to be met effectively like:

- Blood glucose is to fall below that of 50mg/dl.
- Liver glycogen is to be 'empty' or low.
- Low blood glucose can result in elevated Glucagon and low insulin level.
- There should not be available abundant gluconeogenic substrate supply.

Here, there is a need to specify that it not rather a question related to being 'out' or 'in' of ketosis. It can actually be termed as a careful, gradual transition, such that the brain gets evenly and constantly fueled. It is quite ideal for the ketones to be produced in smaller quantities from the levels of blood glucose by about 60mg/dl. It is only when there exist greater ketones concentrations than glucose within the blood that we can consider ourselves to be in ketosis.

In reality, people and more especially the weight trainers are required to consume plenty of glucose on a regular basis for several decades. The liver is just a perfect cable to produce ketones. However, the gluconeogenic pathways that are highly efficient are found to maintain normal low blood glucose just above ketogenic threshold.

The other fact is to be considered that people in huge numbers are seen to be partially insulin resistant. They may have increased fasting insulin (with the upper end of normal range). The small blood glucose amount from gluconeogenesis may induce a good amount of insulin to release for blunting out the output of glucagon as well as to produce ketones.

Sudden deprivation of glucose is likely to have its own consequence, which initially can be a weakness, hunger, lethargy, etc. in many people until there is achieved ketosis. Again, ketosis is not likely to be reached unless the liver gets compelled to leave with gluconeogenesis, to start producing ketones. With proper dietary protein, the liver is likely to continue producing glucose, but not ketones. It is for this reason, no high protein, carb diets are considered to be ketogenic.

Why is Ketosis regarded to be great?

Several cool things take place as the body switches to running mainly on ketones.

- There is a substantial reduction of lipolysis (breakdown of body fat).
- Substantial reduction in muscle catabolism (loss of muscles).
- Maintenance of energy levels in the stable and high state.
- There is noticed elimination of subcutaneous fluid (meaning water retention).

Basically, during ketosis period, our body makes use of fat (ketones) for fueling everything. Hence, muscles are not broken down for deriving glucose. This effectively means that the muscles are spared since it does not offer anything. What the body needs to a great extent is fat. For any dieter, this will mean less loss of muscles than what is exactly achievable through other diet forms.

Besides this, ketones are known to yield just 7 calories/gram. It is much higher when compared to equal glucose mass, however, substantially less (in fact about 22%) than the fat of 9 calorie gram from where it is derived from. Metabolic inefficiencies such as this are preferred. This means, more consumption is possible, but the calories are not derived from the body.

Cooler is the fact that it is not possible for the ketones to be converted into fatty acids. Any excess noticed is excreted by the body through urine. There is likely to be more urine, reduction in muscle glycogen, as well as low aldosterone and low insulin, all of which will equate towards massive excretion of extracellular and intra fluid. This means, well defined, hard muscularity and visible, quick results!

With regards to energy, our brain seriously prefers ketones. Hence, when in ketosis, we have that 'fantastic' feeling, become more positive, alert and clear headed. Since there is never noticed fat shortage for supplying ketones, the energy is always high. You also tend to sleep less and still wake up completely refreshed during ketosis period.

Performing it correctly

For getting into ketosis:

- Intake of carbohydrate is to be zero or nil.
- Intake of protein needs to be low - maximum to about 25% of calories.
- Fat is to account for just 75%+ of the calorie amount.

With low insulin and calories at or probably below maintenance, it is not possible for dietary fat to be deposited within the adipose tissues. Protein being low-ish will mean that the gluconeogenesis is likely to prove quickly to be inadequate for maintaining blood glucose. Hence, irrespective of the body liking it or not, fat is still present to be burnt.

High dietary fat gets oxidized in the normal fashion for cellular energy, however, winds up creating up Acetyl-CoA in huge quantities which tend to exceed TCA cycle capacity. Ketogenesis is considered to be the significant result, which is perhaps, ketones synthesis from excess Acetyl-CoA. When stated in lay terms, higher intake of fat "compels" the body for ketosis. It is how "it is performed correctly".

There are few thoughts that you assumed to be true about fats are to be permanently eliminated. Firstly, fat is not likely to make you become fat. The information that you find in abundance about saturated fats and the evils surrounding it, is quite disproportionate or just wrong. It becomes doubly inapplicable especially when on a ketogenic diet. Ketosis is likely to zoom by saturated fats. At the same time, your heart is also likely to become much better and there will not be noticed any reduction in insulin sensitivity since there is present no insulin around.

Technically speaking, it is not at all essential for maintaining absolute low protein or zero carbs once in ketosis. In case, you desire to reap the rewards, it is termed to be better. Besides, you could be training very hard and eager to follow the cyclic ketogenic diet. Here, you are required to consume fruits, carbs, and others every one to two weeks.

"Performing it right" does not actually make ketogenic dieting to be termed as fun or easy for culinary acrobats, something that should not be mistaken. Probably, they are considered to be among the most restrictive diets that can be used and not termed to be another option present, if animal products are not preferred. You are to come out of the nutritional almanac and simply work out with "20:0:80 protein: carb: fat" diet. This may, however, sound to be somewhat boring.

Supplementation

Several supplements exist which when carefully selected and taken can help the ketogenic diets to be made much more effective and efficient. But in the process, the different popular supplements are likely to be wasted. Overview of the important ones:

ALA and Chromium, although not insulin 'mimickers' like it is claimed, help to improve the sensitivity of insulin, thus resulting in higher glucagon, low insulin levels, quick getting into deeper ketosis.

Again, creatine is found to be somewhat of a waste, with 30% being taken up by muscles. Without glycogen, they cannot be 'volumised' meaningfully.

If HMB works, then it can be regarded to be a wonderful supplement to minimize catabolic period just before achieving ketosis.

Carnitine in Acetyl-L or L from is an important supplement for such type of diets. L-Carnitine is important for forming ketones within the liver.

The other one is Tribulus that is just fabulous and is highly recommended since it helps to magnify the enhanced output of testosterone in the ketogenic diet.

Glutamine is a free-form, branched chain and essential amino that are necessary for both post and pre training. However, this is not to be overdone, since gluconeogenesis is supported.

Also, are found to be important and useful is the ECA Stack fat burners. Forget about HCA inclusion.

Although flaxseed oil is found to be great, there is no need for you to derive 50% of the calories from the essential fatty acids. Only 1% to 10% of calories can be termed to be more than enough.

At the same time, whey protein is termed to be optional. Plenty of protein is not desired.

It is good to have non-carbohydrate soluble fiber supplement. Walnuts can be much easier.

Overall, ketogenic diets do offer plenty of unique benefits which simply cannot be ignored, in case, the ultimate physique or low body fat figure is being pursued. But they are not to be seen as user diet friendly and middle ground compromise that you might prefer since it will be just worst. The choice that you have to make is either perform them right or simply avoid them completely and nothing in-between.

Chapter 4
Difficulties you will face

Your body generally breaks down carbohydrates and uses them as energy. With time, the body tends to build up a good amount of enzymes that are prepared for this particular process. There are present just few enzymes to deal with fats and for storing purpose.

If your body is required to deal with all suddenly increase in fats and lack of glucose, this will mean trying to create new enzyme supply. With your body getting induced into a state of ketogenic, it is likely to use naturally whatever is left of the glucose. This also means that the body will get depleted of the glycogen levels found in the muscles. This will cause lack of energy as well as create general lethargy in the person.

During the initial week, people in huge numbers have reported mental fogginess, headaches, aggravation and dizziness. This can be the result of the electrolytes flushed out since ketosis is known to have a diuretic effect. There is a need to ensure that you consume plenty of water, as well as keep up sodium intake.

As a matter of fact, with salt, your should try to go overboard, since salt means everything. Water retention is possible with sodium and it also assists to replenish the electrolytes. This temporary feeling of grogginess, for the majority, is considered to be the biggest danger that anyone is likely to face. This is known as the "Keto Flu".

Know the common side effects

Some of the common side effects noticed upon starting keto are given below. The issues are said to relate frequently to lack of vitamins (micronutrients) or dehydration in the body. There is a need to ensure that sufficient water is being consumed every day amounting to about gallon a day, as well as consuming food with plenty of micronutrient sources.

Cramps

Specifically, leg cramps are quite common when beginning with ketogenic diet. Usually, it occurs during the night or morning time and is regarded by the experts to be a trivial issue. It is rather seen to be a sign that the body does have a lack of minerals, more specifically magnesium.

Plenty of fluid is to be consumed. Salt is to be had with food. Doing so is likely to help tackle magnesium loss and to eliminate such issues. In case, the problem is still found to persist, then supplement with a magnesium supplement.

Constipation

Constipation is often caused due to dehydration. The simple solution that can be offered to take care of this situation is to increase the amount of water intake. One should have at least gallon of water in a day. Also, the vegetables with fibers can help a lot. Good quality fiber is to be derived from the non-starchy vegetables that can prove to be more than useful to eliminate this problem. If more is required for treating this issue, then psyllium husk powder is sure to work. Also probiotic can be effective.

Heart palpitations

While transitioning to keto, the heart is likely to beat much harder and faster. This is quite the norm and hence, there is nothing to worry about the same. But if the problem is seen to still persist, then there is a genuine need to drink plenty of fluid and to take sufficient salt in food. It is sufficient for eliminating the issue immediately. Potassium supplement when taken once in a day can also help.

Reduced physical performance

Some limitations can be noticed on the performances upon beginning the keto diet. However, this is generally from the body that tries to adapt using fat. With the body starts to make use of fat for deriving energy, all the endurance and strength is likely to return back to normalcy. If still performance related problems are being noticed, then intake of carbs before the workout is likely to prove to be more than beneficial.

Know the less-commonly noticed keto diet side effects

There are also noticed some less common problems upon starting a keto diet. Some of these are said to be related to micronutrients and hydration. Experts recommend drinking water in good quantities and to replenish the electrolytes.

Hair loss

If hair loss is being experienced within five months of initiating this diet process, then it is just a temporary phase. You can have multivitamins and carry out your normal life. Although keto diet does not involve hair loss side effects, it can be minimized by ensuring that the calories are not restricted upon excessively. Also, there is a genuine need to get minimum night sleep of eight hours.

Breastfeeding

Several mixed and matched results have emerged relating keto and breastfeeding. Presently, nothing is found to be well researched on this particular subject. It is found that ketogenic diets are healthy to be practiced when breastfeeding. 30 to 50g of extra carbs is to be added from fruits while breastfeeding. This can help the body to produce more milk that is beneficial for the baby. Extra calories are also required to be added. Milk production can be improved with the extra fat of about 300 to 500 calories. But before starting, it will be wise to contact the experienced and qualified medical professional.

Increased cholesterol

It is usually noticed to be a wonderful thing. There are several studies that have been pointing towards the elevation of cholesterol while practicing low carb keto diet. It is because of the increase in good cholesterol (HDL) that reduces the chances of catching heart diseases. Also, are witnessed increased triglyceride counts. However, it is seen to be something common among people trying to lose weight. But the increases are likely to subside with normalization of weight loss.

Some percentage of people is likely to experience increased LDL cholesterol. Such elevated levels usually are fine, although they are tough to test. LDL cholesterol does come with its own dangers, is because of the density and size that are displayed to be healthy on the keto diet.

Gallstones

When gallstones and keto are concerned, many people have witnessed complete curing or improvement in gallstone problems. However, the downside is that there have been reports of an increase in discomfort upon starting with low carb. By sticking to it, vast improvement can be experienced. The other question that is commonly asked with regards to gallstones like, "Is it possible to initiate keto, if the gallbladder is removed?" The experts conclude that it will not be a problem. Probably, you may be eager to improve gradually your fat, thus allowing your system with some precious time for getting used to it.

Keto rash

No scientific explanation or reasoning exists as to why some people may develop itching upon starting a keto diet. It is probably irritation caused from the acetone, which is excreted with sweat. It is always better and wise to check out the clothing options so as to wick or absorb sweat from the body. At the same time, it also will be worth going for a shower immediately after the activity causing sweat is undertaken. If it is found to be a lasting issue, causing problems, then upping the carbs or simply changing the exercise plans is recommended!

Indigestion

Switching to a keto diet, generally speaking, is said to eliminate heartburn and indigestion. It is important to note that few people may experience increased attacks as they start out for the first time. If problems are being experienced, then it will be wise to simply limit the fat intake amount and to increase gradually this amount that is taken per day in two week period.

Dangers of starting keto diet

Can production of ketone in the body become too high? The experts conclude that it is a possible and such state is known as ketoacidosis. It is not, however, likely under the normal circumstances. For the majority, it is just a challenge to get into the optimal ranges to be in ketosis. You are not likely to be in a territory requiring medical intervention. Type 1 diabetics are regarded to be the main exception for ketoacidosis. This may take place if the levels of insulin are found to be severely low, something that is very rare in a person having normal functioning of the pancreas. Again, dangerously high levels of ketone may result in secretion of insulin.

There are indeed several misconceptions that exist with regards to low carb dieting that is said to have caused this infamous outlook on a ketogenic diet. Numerous studies have been conducted on this type of diet for more than three decades and it has been found that fat in higher amounts and few carbs definitely are beneficial.

At times, people tend to mix keto with that of high carb, high-fat diets that are disastrous for the body. It is quite obvious that upon consuming a good amount of fatty foods, rich in sugar, you are likely to be in trouble.

Planning to go on a low-fat diet! Studies have shown that keto diet is not only effective when compared to low-fat dieting, but also is a healthier option to select. While consuming foods that are high in fat and carbohydrates, your body will be producing glucose naturally. The human body does find carbohydrate to be the easiest element to be processed. Hence, it is likely to use them first, thus resulting in excess storage of fat immediately. This, in turn, causes a gain in weight along with other types of health problems which are associated with the presence of high fat and high carbohydrate diets, but not keto.

Hence, as a precaution, there is a genuine need to check with the qualified physician about all concerns that may emerge when starting on the keto diet. It is important to be wary of if any medications are being taken for treating pre-existing medical conditions. In such a case, extra monitoring is necessary. Again when breastfeeding, be careful, as there will be required increase in carb intake.

Chapter 5
How to overcome them

The truth is that ketogenic low-carbohydrate diets have proved to become popular among people across the globe with time. They are regarded very highly in many circles and found to be maintainable, effective weight loss diets.

Some tips to optimize success on ketogenic diet

- Consume plenty of water: When on a keto diet, the body is likely to have a tough time trying to retain water as it requires. Therefore, staying hydrated all the time is necessary. Experts are of the opinion that women should consume beverage of about 2.2 liters and men around 3 liters on a daily basis. The urine's color is considered to be an excellent indicator of practicing proper hydration. It is essential to have a water bottle handy when going outside.
- Remember the fat: Fuel is required by our body for proper functioning. Upon limiting intake of carbohydrate, especially to such a level where ketosis is induced, our bodies require an alternative source of fuel. Our bodies get converted into fat since protein is found to be a poor energy source. Any fat that is consumed when in ketosis is said to be used for energy, thus making it quite difficult for storing fat during this period. It is important to select unsaturated, healthy fats, which can be derived in foods like olives, avocados, seeds and nuts.

- Identify the carb limit: Not every person has the same type of body. Few dieters may want to adhere to low carb strict diet and consume lesser carbs in a day by about 20 gms. The others may find it cool to consume carbohydrates by about 50, 75 and 100 gm. Trial and error method is undoubtedly the best way to find out what suits best. Any ketone urinalysis strip brand can be purchased to identify the carbohydrate limit. If there is found some wiggle room, then sticking to the diet will become much easier.
- Choose liquor wisely: In keto diet, you are free to drink liquor, but without damaging your weight loss course of action. Unsweetened liquors like rum, vodka, gin, tequila, scotch, whiskey, brandy, and cognac are permitted combined with low carb beer. You can drink sufficient amount of water and low carb mixers for staying hydrated. When in ketosis, hangovers can be real bad. Calories do count! So you should stay within the limit.
- Be patient: Keto diet is popular for offering quick weight loss remedy. During the diet's early stage, loss of weight is seen to be a time consuming, slow process. Hence, it will not be wise to just freak out, if weight loss is not experienced or for few days, slight weight increase is noticed. The weight of the body is likely to vary from one day to the other as well as throughout the day. This is based on several factors. Metrics are to be used for the body measurements or how the clothes fit. This way, the progress made can be noticed.

Precautions to be taken when on keto diet and some frequently asked questions

This type of diet tends to focus on calories derived from protein and fat and avoiding carbohydrates. As carbs are absent, the body tends to make use of protein and fats for deriving energy. This diet is named for ketone bodies which are actually waste products from fat breakdown. They can be measured through urine. The applications tend to include neurological disorder treatment and weight loss, though the dietary specifics could be substantially different between the applications. This diet is considered to be extreme and also can prove to be termed as a potent stressor for the body. It needs to be pursued with great caution, under the supervision of the local physician and with proper knowledge and understanding.

Does it really help to control seizures?

Some seizure disorders like epilepsy may occur if the brain activity is noticed to be out of control occasionally, thus resulting in a cluster of uncontrolled movements, behavior, and sensations. This diet is found to be quite effective to control seizures, which were found to be untreatable by the other forms of treatments. The ketogenic diet is said to mimic starvation to help control the seizures, the functioning something that is not yet understood. During the manifestation of ketogenic diet exclusively for epilepsy, over 80% of the daily calories is said to be derived from fat.

Can this work for Tourette's?

It is a neurological disorder syndrome that is defined by repetitive, uncontrollable sounds or movements called tics. Evidence state energy metabolism's role is to regulate specific neurotransmitter level to control brain activity level. But the diet's effectiveness towards controlling syndrome tics of Tourette is not yet determined.

47

Can the diet help to prevent kidney stones?

The fact is that kidney stones form accumulated mineral deposits which are to be passed painfully through the urinary tract, so as to be eliminated from the body. The kidney stones are considered to be the diet's occasional side effect. The overall health of the person is quite important that the diet prevents kidney stones.

Does the diet help to raise blood cholesterol?

Since this diet is found to be high in fat, probably you might wonder if it raises blood cholesterol. But, the diet comprising of about 61% of fat-lowered blood cholesterol including that of triglycerides. Saturated fats are known to significantly contribute to the blood cholesterol levels. The diet that is high in saturated fats is likely to raise levels of cholesterol. It will be wise to avoid those unhealthy foods that are high in saturated fats, when on a ketogenic diet.

Does it cause insulin resistance?

Direct nutrients, more especially the sugar glucose are helped by the hormone insulin into the body's cells. One of the initial steps towards several diseases like metabolic syndrome and Type II diabetes is insulin resistance. According to a study conducted found that when lab mice had been fed with ketogenic diet had developed in their livers, insulin resistance. Another study found that reduction of overall insulin resistance was found among humans upon starting ketogenic diet. Human trials were said to involve men not having pre-diabetes or Type 2 diabetes signs.

Does it make the hair to grow?

Few benefits derived from this diet may arise from the hormonal level effects as well as gene expression. They may vary between one individual and the other. At the same time, hormone testosterone is likely to alter hair development. But the diet's effects on testosterone level are seen to be unclear. Studies found that testosterone level among healthy men was not affected by low carb diet. If any abnormal hair loss or growth is experienced when on a ketogenic diet, then it will be wise to consult the qualified physician.

Does it include dairy?

The fact is dairy is said to be rich in protein and fats and also low in carbs. This can be stapled food when on a keto diet. Dairy along with meats do offer a wonderful source of fat and protein that is required on the diet without actually risking getting plenty of carbs. Moreover, high-fat dairy like heavy cream is used for calories especially on a ketogenic diet.

Is sweet potato allowed to be consumed?

They are said to have huge amounts of carbohydrate in them. Hence, they are better avoided or intake limited when on a keto diet, which limits carbs severely. When on a diet for losing weight, you can consume sweet potatoes in moderation. However, take note that keto diet is rather a low carb diet and not any no-carb diet. Epilepsy is treated with extreme keto diet to derive calories from carbs in 5% to 10%. Most of the carbs during the keto diet is to be derived mainly from fresh vegetables.

Is it possible to consume whole grain bread?

It is made of carbohydrate primarily. Even though carbs are absorbed more slowly when compared to white bread, this is to be avoided when on a ketogenic diet. If the desire is to lose weight, then whole grain bread can be consumed within 2 hours of finishing the workout. It is during this period that the body gets optimized for replenishing the glycogen in the liver and muscles.

How long to pursue ketogenic diet?

The keto diet needs to be short term plan if the desire is for losing weight. Substantial weight loss can be experienced by the majority of the people within 4-6 weeks of initiating this plan. The diet, when practiced for 8-12 weeks, is likely to reduce greatly body fat, if the willpower is present for overcoming the loss of energy, cravings and mood disturbances. For treating epilepsy and various types of disorders, the diet is to be practiced for an indefinite period, however, under the strict medical supervision and consultation of the experienced and qualified physician. Such diets are customized personally by the nutritionist and the physician to suit your body needs and requirements and to do away with all negative aspects.

Chapter 6
Results & Testimonies

There are hundreds of testimonials that have been put up by people, especially those who have benefitted immensely from following a ketogenic diet. This diet has been found to be really wonderful and recommended to the others, who are eager to shed excess weight and enjoy having a normal, slim body.

- Michelle is 30 years old and had struggled a lot throughout her life with her weight. Growing up heavy indeed was quite hard for her. She was the talk of the school among her friends and even teachers, which made to lose her self-esteem. As she reached middle school, she had to wear clothing for grown-up women, which she felt really miserable. This only continued with time and there was no respite for her, although she had tried out various activities to reduce her weight. It is at that point of time that she came across keto diet and some recommended exercise regimen that she took up seriously. Her lifestyle changed for the better. She saw changes in her body weight and now is enjoying her life just like the others.
- Ronald Robinson and his wife had lost combined 100 lbs through keto diet. Cutting out the carbs from the diet was really terrifying in the initial stage. Some research on keto diet did help to boost his morale and convince him and his wife to pursue it to lose weight. They cooked the keto recipes that they found on the web and changed their lifestyle

for the better. Their favorite recipe was between buttermilk pancakes and low carb bacon meatloaf. But they had to forgo the pancakes. Coconut flour was the favorite ingredient used for preparing the keto recipes. Their motivation was their daughter. She was a real morale booster, especially when energy is concerned. They were able to overcome all hassles that they faced with strong determination.

There are much more testimonials on the web that will not only favor and prompt you to perform keto diet but also recommend you and the others to start it immediately without any delay.

Recipes

Some tasty recipes of ketogenic diet dishes.

What can I consume when on a keto diet?

This is a question that is commonly asked by people especially those who are interested in going on a keto diet. It is important to plan in advance the menu. A viable diet strategy is what is required, so that it followed rigorously, to achieve the desired objectives. What is to be consumed will depend upon how quickly you desire to be in this keto state. The much more restrictive you find yourself on carbohydrates, which is to be lesser than 15 grams in a day, the much faster are you to enter ketosis.

If you are eager to restrict your intake of carbohydrates then consider taking vegetables, dairy, and nuts. Avoid consuming refined carbohydrates like wheat (cereals, pasta, bread), starch (legumes, beans, potatoes) or fruit. However, some minor exceptions to the above include berries, star fruit, and avocado that can be eaten in moderation.

What is to be avoided?

- Sugar – maple syrup, agave, honey, etc.
- Grains – cereal, rice, corn, wheat, etc.
- Tubers – yams, potato, etc.
- Fruit – oranges, bananas, apples, etc.

What is recommended?

- Leafy greens: kale, spinach, etc.
- Meats: eggs, poultry, lamb, beef, fish, etc.
- Vegetables found in the ground – cauliflower, broccoli, etc.
- Seeds and nuts – sunflower seeds, walnuts, macadamias, etc.
- Dairy having high-fat content – butter, high fat cream, hard cheeses, etc.
- Berries and avocado – low-glycemic impact berries, blackberries, raspberries, etc.
- Sweeteners – low carb sweeteners, monk fruit, erythritol, stevia, etc.
- Other types of fats – saturated fats, high-fat salad dressing, coconut oil, etc.

There is a need to understand that keto is quite high in fat, low in carbs and moderate in protein. The intake of nutrients is to be somewhat like this:

- Carbohydrate – 5%
- Protein - 25%
- Fats – 70%

For everyday dieting, typically around 20 to 30 gram of net carb has been recommended. However, the much lower the glucose and carb level intake, the much better can the results be expected. If keto is being practiced for weight loss, then it will be a great idea to keep proper track of both the net carbs and total carbs.

It is important to consume protein always as required with fat trying to fill up the rest of the calories that are required every day. Net carbs are actually the total dietary carbohydrates, less the total fiber. The total carbs recommended should be below 35g, while net carbs are to be below 25g.

In case, you feel hungry at any point of time, then you can select cheese, peanut butter, seeds and nuts for curbing your appetite. During the long term, snacking is likely to slow down weight loss, something that you need to keep an eye upon. At times, the need for snacks with that of the meal is often confused upon.

Including vegetables in keto diet

Leafy and dark green vegetables have always been a wonderful choice. The meals should mostly comprise of protein coming from vegetables along with some fat. If you are a non-vegetarian, then chicken breast that is basted with olive oil and combined with cheese and broccoli is sure to do the trick. The steak that is topped with butter knob and side of spinach which is sautéed with olive oil is just perfect.

There are varieties of delicious vegetables readily available in the market to be purchased and consumed. When net carb is concerned, for example, one cup of broccoli,

- There are 6 grams of carbohydrates in one cup in total.
- Also is present 2 grams of fiber in one cup
- Hence, 6 grams of total carbs is taken and dietary fiber of 2 grams is subtracted.
- It is likely to give out the net carbs which in this case is f 4 grams.

My top 7 keto/low carb recipes

There are indeed several low carb keto recipes that can be found to be mouth-watering and tempting. They can be prepared to be consumed by people of all ages. There are recipes that can be had repeatedly, without you feeling bored. They are just delicious every time you have it and are likely to compel you to have more of it. Irrespective of you leading in a keto lifestyle or eager to try out some delicious food, the recipes mentioned below are sure to satisfy your cravings and hunger. They also good for your health and keep you physically and mentally fit.

- For the initial week of being on a keto diet, you can prepare a meal that you can always have whenever you are hungry. This is a recipe that not only you're but also your friends are sure to love consuming it. The combination of butter and sauce can seem to be quite incredible, such that you are sure to have it on all the meals that you have, even on the salads. Bacon grease can also be put in salads, something you are sure to enjoy.
- The keto diet can comprise of veggies and fruits. Cutting them every time can be a horrifying experience during the initial days. But with your taste bud slowly adapting to the change, you are sure to appreciate the sweetness of berries. Moreover, cutting sugar tends to bring out subtle sweetness as well as flavors among all foods. The truth is that blueberries can be real sweet and tasty, such that sugar will no longer be required by many. These muffins can be made at least once in a month to be consumed. The tip here to make it all the tastier will be to add butter along with a dash of cinnamon or nutmeg.
- When veggie is concerned, you can introduce celeriac root. If you not have heard about it, then simply Google it and you are likely to come across a whole lot of information about the same. When on a keto diet, you can use it for pasta. You can always have one in your fridge and use it for pasta and fries including bacon as well as celery root egg skillet. It is a wonderful dish that is sure to satisfy and also overall all of your pasta mouth requirements.
- Chocolate pudding is a real delight that is sure to be savored by everyone and loved by all ages. You can

have pudding created and simply add some dark beer into the preparation.

- Another recipe that you can brag about with your friends and colleagues and prepare when the air around is still chilly is the chai that is fondled with coconut milk. It can turn out to be a real sweet earthy bliss.

- The chocolate covered maple bacon is simply another recipe that does deserve a second look. you can use bacon grease for preparing the chocolate.

- You can also brine your chicken well within pickle juice and simply wonder how to consume it. It is so delicious and moist that you will simply excuse yourself to have the chicken strips placed into plastic baggies filled with pickle juice without any delay. You can also fry them in the pork rinds.

Conclusion

Overall, the ketogenic diet is just fabulous for those who are eager to shed their excess weight and appear slim and trim, with a beautiful personality and look, just like their favorite Hollywood stars and celebrities. This type of diet does require you to be disciplined and follow a strict regimen, to avoid all types of temptation, so as to derive the desired results. You can rest assured that by consulting the physician and nutritional expert from time to time, the results are likely to be achieved without experiencing any kind of side effects. At the same time, this type of diet is extremely safe to be followed and is also cost effective. There are present numerous keto diet recipes on the web that can be accessed and followed on a regular basis.

Thankyou For Reading

If you enjoyed this book or received value from it in any way, then I'd like to ask you for a favor: would you be kind enough to leave a review for this book on Amazon? It'd be greatly appreciated!